RENAL DIET COOKBOOK FOR STAGE 4

NUTRIENT RECIPES FOR YOUR KIDNEYS AND WELL-BEING

SHAUVE RIVK

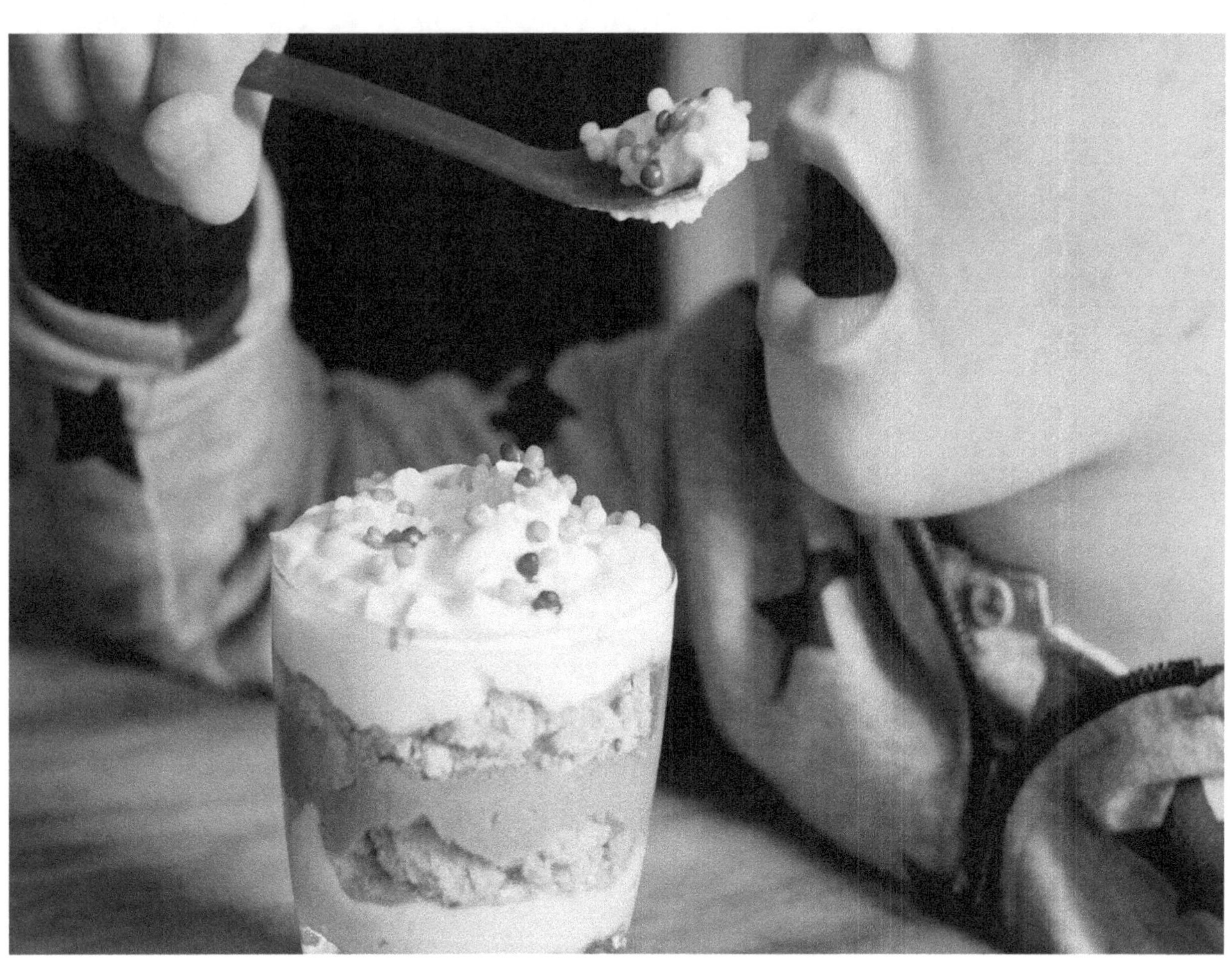

CONTENTS

☐ <u>CONCLUSION</u>

INTRODUCTION

Hello and thank you for visiting "Renal Diet Cookbook For Stage 4: Nutrient Recipes For Your Kidneys And Well-being." This cookbook is more than simply a collection of recipes; it is a road map to greater health, a higher quality of life, and a brighter future for those with stage 4 renal disease. Living with chronic kidney disease may be difficult, and finding the appropriate balance in your diet can help you manage your symptoms and reduce the course of the condition. That is why we produced this cookbook to offer you wholesome and tasty dishes adapted to the specific dietary demands of people with stage 4 renal disease.

We recognize that dealing with a significant health condition may be overwhelming and that adopting dietary adjustments can be difficult. This cookbook is here to help you by giving you the information, resources, and motivation you need to take charge of your health and flourish despite your diagnosis. The dishes in this cookbook are kidney-friendly, which means they are low in sodium, potassium, and phosphorus, and they are also high in nutrients that are needed for overall health. We carefully picked foods recognized for their health advantages, and we created dishes that are not only nutritious but also delicious and filling.

This cookbook has varieties of recipes for breakfast, soups, salads, main entrees, side dishes, and even desserts. You will find something to fit your interests and needs, whether you are seeking quick and easy dinners for busy weeknights or exceptional delicacies to enjoy with loved ones.

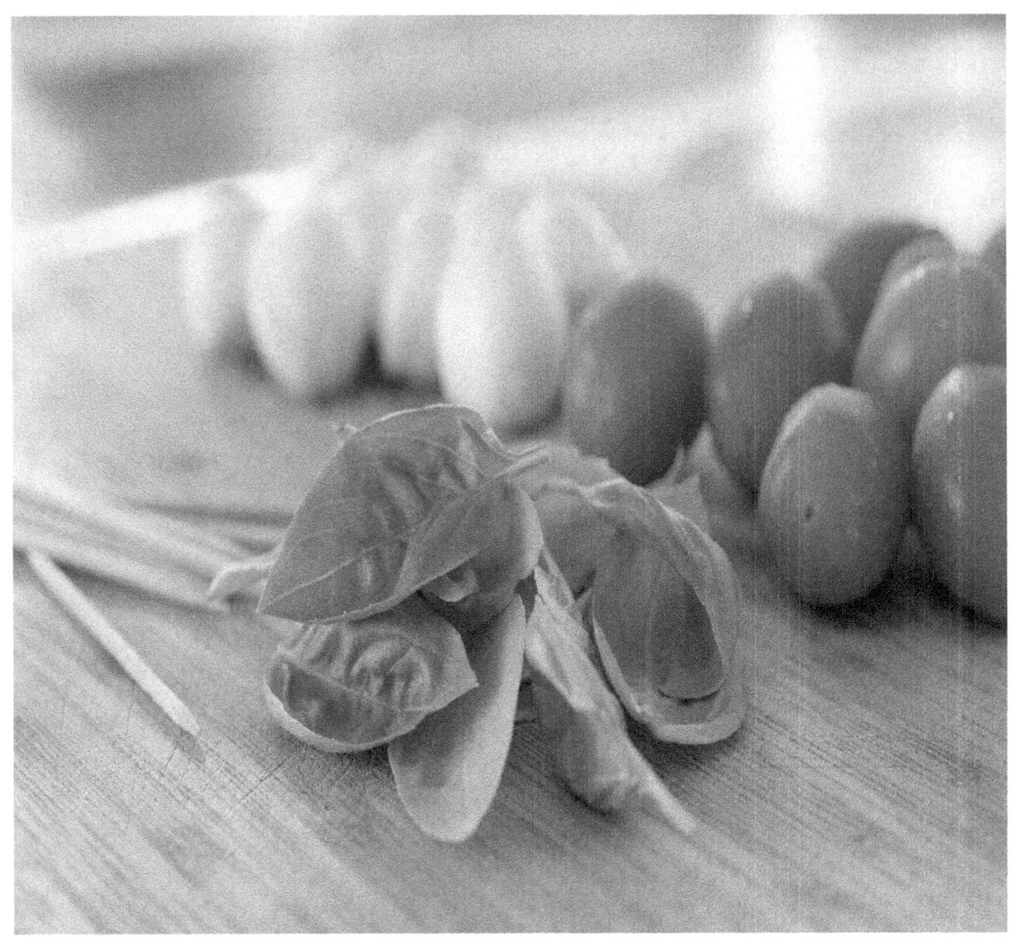

This cookbook, however, is more than just a compilation of recipes. It is also a resource for learning about the dietary requirements of people with stage 4 renal disease. We give clear and comprehensive information on the role of nutrition in renal disease management, as well as practical suggestions and guidance on how to make healthy food choices and prepare balanced meals.

We think that food should be a source of joy and sustenance, and we are devoted to assisting you in rediscovering the enjoyment of eating while dealing with the obstacles of renal illness. We put our hearts and souls into this cookbook, and we hope it will become a valued companion on your road to greater health and well-being. So, why should you waste time buying this book? The solution is straightforward: your health and happiness are worth it. This cookbook is a lifeline, a source of support and information that may help you take charge of your health and live your best life, even if you have a significant health condition.

The dishes in this cookbook are not only tasty and filling, but they are also particularly intended to promote kidney health and general well-being. You may help to slow the course of your kidney disease, control your symptoms, and improve your quality of life by following the suggestions and recipes in this cookbook. However, the advantages of this diet extend beyond the physical. Cooking and eating excellent, nutritional meals may also improve your mental and emotional health. Even in bad circumstances, it may bring a sense of accomplishment and fulfillment, as well as a source of comfort and pleasure.

We think that everyone deserves to eat well and be healthy, and we are dedicated to providing you with the tools and resources you need to do so.

Whether you've recently been diagnosed with kidney disease or have been dealing with it for years, this cookbook is here to help and empower you to take charge of your health and your life. Start your journey to greater health, a higher quality of life, and a brighter future. Your health and well-being are important to us, and we will be there for you every step of the way.

ONE

THE IMPORTANCE OF NUTRITION IN KIDNEY DISEASE MANAGEMENT

Nutrition is critical in the treatment of renal disease. The appropriate diet can help reduce disease development, control symptoms, and enhance overall quality of life. Finding the correct balance in your diet, on the other hand, can be difficult, especially when coping with the unique dietary limitations that come with stage 4 renal disease. That is why we developed this cookbook. We recognize the difficulties associated with treating renal illness, so we've carefully designed recipes that are low in sodium, potassium, and phosphorus while being high in nutrients that promote kidney health. We've also included clear and straightforward information about the role of nutrition in kidney disease management, so you can make informed food choices and prepare balanced meals that benefit your health.

THE IMPORTANCE OF MAKING HEALTHY FOOD CHOICES

Making appropriate eating choices is important for controlling renal illness, but it may also improve your mental and emotional well-being. Even in tough circumstances, cooking and eating good, wholesome meals may bring a sense of accomplishment and fulfillment, as well as a source of comfort and enjoyment. That's why we've included recipes for everything from morning meals to soups, salads, main entrees, side dishes, and desserts in this handbook. Whether you're searching for quick and simple weekday dinners or exceptional delicacies to share with family and friends, you'll find something to fit your interests and requirements.

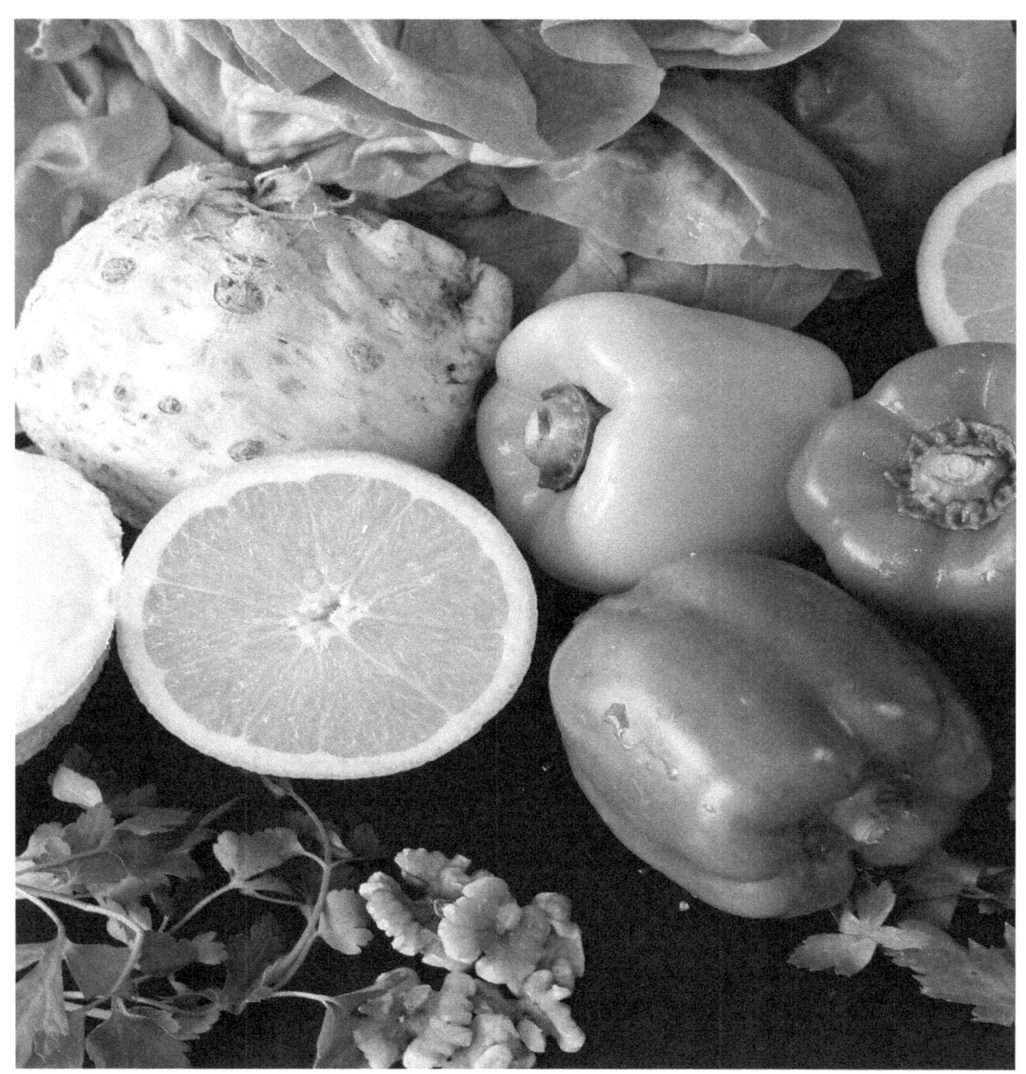

HOW THIS COOKBOOK CAN SUPPORT YOU

Remember, this cookbook serves as a guide, companion, and source of support for those with stage 4 renal disease. We understand the difficulties that come with treating renal illness, and we're here to help you every step of the way. You can take charge of your health and flourish despite your diagnosis by following the directions and recipes in this cookbook. Even while you negotiate the obstacles of renal illness, you'll learn how to make smart food choices, prepare balanced meals that support your health, and rediscover the pleasure of eating.

So, why bother? Your health and well-being are worth it, and we're here to help you along the journey.

TWO

GETTING STARTED: UNDERSTANDING THE DIETARY NEEDS OF INDIVIDUALS WITH STAGE 4 KIDNEY DISEASE

Nutrition is critical in the treatment of stage 4 renal disease. The appropriate diet can help reduce disease development, control symptoms, and enhance overall quality of life. Finding the correct balance in your diet, on the other hand, can be difficult, especially when coping with the unique dietary limitations that come with stage 4 renal disease. In this chapter, we'll look at the dietary demands of people with stage 4 renal disease and provide you with the knowledge you need to make informed food choices and prepare balanced meals that will benefit your health and well-being.

THE ROLE OF SODIUM, POTASSIUM, AND PHOSPHORUS IN KIDNEY HEALTH

When it comes to controlling renal illness, three crucial minerals to remember are salt, potassium, and phosphorus. These nutrients are essential for maintaining fluid balance, neuron function, and bone health, but in excess, they can be detrimental, especially for people with renal disease. In this part, we'll look at the function of sodium, potassium, and phosphorus in kidney health and give you practical advice on how to manage your intake of these nutrients to improve your health and well-being.

Sodium is a mineral that aids in fluid equilibrium, neuron function, and muscle function. Excess salt consumption, on the other hand, can cause high blood pressure, which is a typical concern for people with renal disease. To control your sodium intake, restrict your intake of processed and packaged foods, which are generally rich in sodium, and season your meals using herbs, spices, and other flavorings rather than salt.

Potassium is yet another necessary mineral that aids in fluid equilibrium, neuron function, and muscle function. Excess potassium consumption, on the other hand, can cause hyperkalemia, a condition defined by high levels of potassium in the blood, which can be dangerous for those with renal disease. To control your potassium intake, restrict your consumption of high-potassium foods like bananas, oranges, and potatoes and instead pick low-potassium choices like apples, grapes, and rice.

Phosphorus is a vital mineral that aids in the formation and maintenance of healthy bones and teeth, as well as the creation of energy in the body. Excess phosphorus consumption, on the other hand, can cause hyperphosphatemia, a condition defined by high amounts of phosphorus in the blood, which can be dangerous for those with renal disease. To control your phosphorus intake, restrict your consumption of high-phosphorus foods like dairy products, nuts, and seeds and instead pick low-phosphorus options like fruits, vegetables, and grains.

TIPS AND STRATEGIES FOR MAKING HEALTHY FOOD CHOICES AND CREATING BALANCED MEALS

Making appropriate eating choices is important for controlling renal illness, but it may also improve your mental and emotional well-being. Even in tough circumstances, cooking and eating good, wholesome meals may bring a sense of accomplishment and fulfillment, as well as a source of comfort and enjoyment. We'll provide you with practical advice and techniques for choosing healthy food choices and preparing balanced meals that will benefit your health and well-being in this part. When it comes to eating healthily, it's crucial to prioritize complete, unprocessed meals like fruits, vegetables, grains, and lean meats. These foods are nutrient-dense and naturally low in sodium, potassium, and phosphorus, making them an excellent choice for those who have renal disease.

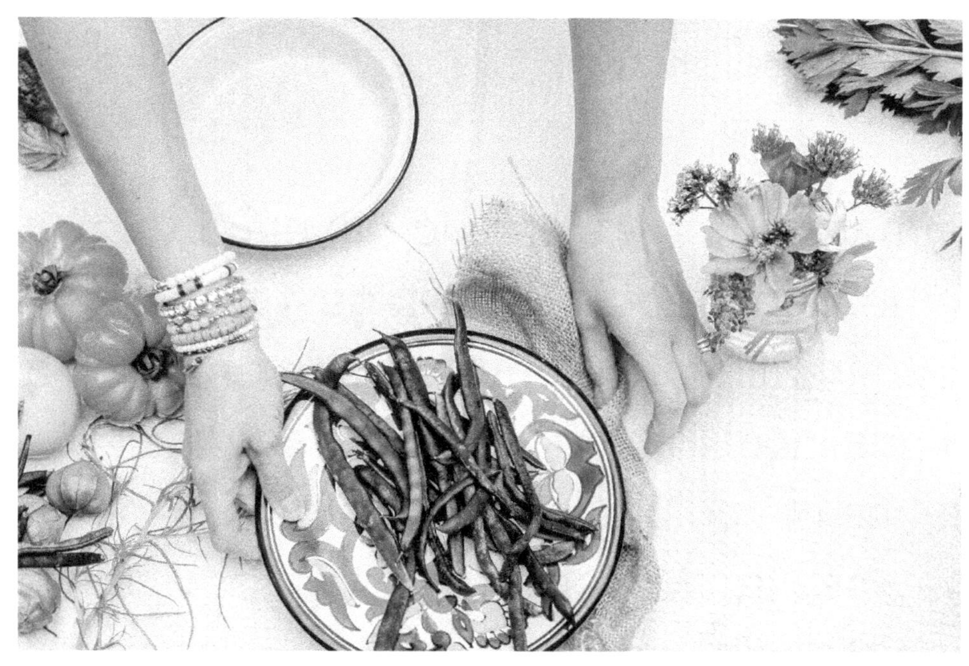

It's also crucial to watch your portion sizes and consume a variety of meals to ensure your body gets all the nutrients it needs. This can help you regulate your salt, potassium, and phosphorus consumption while also supporting your general health and well-being. It is critical to incorporate a range of dietary categories while preparing balanced meals, such as fruits, vegetables, grains, and lean meats. This can help you receive a variety of nutrients while also supporting your health and well-being. It's also vital to watch portion sizes and pick foods low in sodium, potassium, and phosphorus.

To summarize, understanding the dietary requirements of people with stage 4 renal disease is critical for treating the condition and enhancing your overall quality of life. We've discussed the importance of sodium, potassium, and phosphorus in kidney health, as well as practical advice and methods for selecting good food choices and preparing balanced meals that promote your health and well-being. So don't put it off any longer. Your health and well-being are worth it, and we're here to help you along the journey.

THREE

BREAKFAST RECIPES

Breakfast is generally referred to as the most important meal of the day, and with good reason. It jump-starts your metabolism, gives you the energy you need to get through the day, and keeps you focused and alert. However, when you have stage 4 kidney disease, it can be difficult to locate breakfast alternatives that are both delicious and kidney-friendly.

In this chapter, we'll look at a range of breakfast recipes that are not only tasty and filling but are also adapted to the specific dietary needs of people with stage 4 renal disease. From Berry and Yogurt Parfait to Quinoa and Berry Breakfast Bowl, these dishes will get your day started correctly.

BERRY AND YOGURT PARFAIT

This Berry and Yogurt Parfait is a quick and easy breakfast that is both tasty and healthy. It's loaded with protein and fiber to keep you full and happy all morning, and it's crafted with layers of creamy yogurt, juicy berries, and crunchy granola.

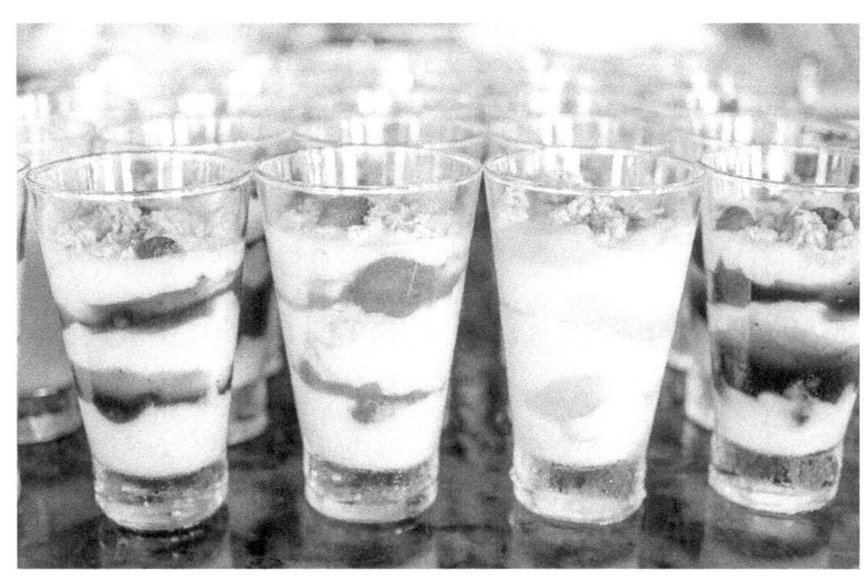

Ingredients:

1 cup plain, low-fat yogurt

1/2 cup fresh berries (strawberries, blueberries, raspberries, etc.)

2 granola tablespoons

Instructions:

Layer 1/3 cup yogurt, 2 tablespoons berries, and 1 tablespoon granola in a glass or container.

Continue layering until all of the ingredients are used.

Serve right away and enjoy!

VEGGIE OMELETTE WITH TOAST

This veggie omelet on toast is a filling breakfast choice that is high in protein and minerals. It's cooked with eggs, veggies, and whole-grain bread, and it's a terrific way to start your day with a nutritious and balanced meal.

Ingredients:

two huge eggs

1/4 cup diced veggies (for example, bell peppers, onions, or spinach)

1 whole-grain bread piece

1 tablespoon of olive oil

Instructions:

Whisk the eggs in a small bowl until fully mixed

Place the olive oil in a nonstick pan or skillet over medium heat

Cook until the veggies are soft, approximately 3-5 minutes

Cook until the eggs are set, about 2–3 minutes, over the veggies

Serve the omelette folded in half with whole-grain bread.

BANANA AND NUT SMOOTHIE

Banana and Nut Smoothie is a light and invigorating breakfast choice that's ideal for a hectic morning. It's created with bananas, almonds, and almond milk and is a terrific way to start your day with a nutritious and tasty smoothie.

Ingredients:

one banana 1/4 cup nuts (almonds, walnuts, cashews, etc.)

1 quart of almond milk

1 teaspoon (optional) honey

Instructions:

Blend the banana, almonds, almond milk, and honey
(if using) in a blender

Blend until the batter or mixture is very smooth and
creamy

Pour into a glass and serve right away.

AVOCADO TOAST WITH EGG

This avocado toast with egg is a quick and easy
breakfast that is ideal for a quiet weekend

morning. It's created with creamy avocado, a fried egg, and whole-grain bread, and it's a terrific way to start your day with a nutritious meal.

Ingredients:

1 whole-grain bread piece

a half avocado

1 big egg

1 tablespoon of olive oil

Season with salt and pepper to taste.

Instructions:

Toast until the bread is golden brown and crunchy

Spread the avocado mash on the bread

Place the olive oil in a nonstick pan or skillet over medium heat

Cook until the whites are firm but the yolk is still runny in the skillet, about 2-3 minutes

Season the egg on top of the avocado toast with salt and pepper

Serve right away and enjoy!

QUINOA AND BERRY BREAKFAST BOWL

Quinoa and Berry Meal Bowl is a filling and healthy meal alternative that is ideal for a hectic morning. It's filled with protein and fiber to keep you full and content all morning, and it's created with cooked quinoa, fresh berries, and a drizzle of honey.

Ingredients:

1 cup quinoa

cooked

1/2 cup fresh berries (strawberries, blueberries, raspberries, etc.)

1 tablespoon of honey

Instructions:

Combine the cooked quinoa, fresh berries, and honey in a mixing dish

Stir until well blended

Serve right away and enjoy!

To summarize, breakfast is an essential meal of the day, and choosing tasty and kidney-friendly alternatives might be difficult. We've looked at a selection of breakfast dishes that are not only delicious and filling but also customized to the specific nutritional needs of people with stage 4 renal disease. From Berry and Yogurt Parfait to Quinoa and Berry Breakfast Bowl, these dishes will get your day started correctly. So don't put it off any longer. Your health and well-being are worth it, and we're here to help you along the journey.

FOUR

SOUP AND SALAD RECIPES

Soups and salads are frequently thought of as light

and refreshing dinner alternatives, but they may also
be heavy and filling.

In this chapter, we'll look at soup and salad recipes
that are not only tasty and savory but also adapted
to the specific nutritional needs of those with stage 4
renal disease. These dishes, ranging from creamy
carrot and ginger soup to mixed green salad with
lemon-tahini dressing, are ideal for a light lunch or a

refreshing dinner. So, let's get started and look at some great kidney-friendly soup and salad dishes!

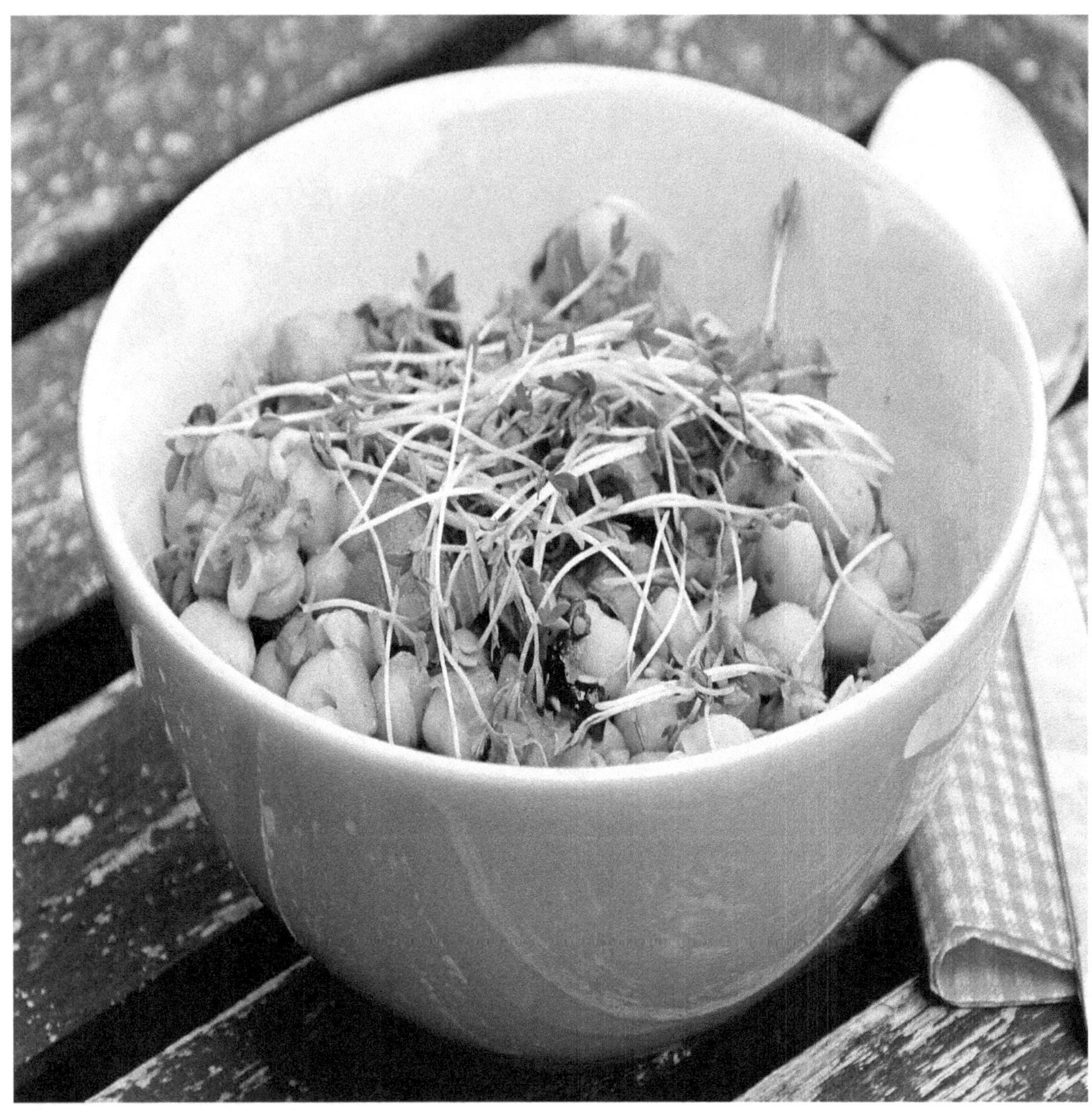

CREAMY CARROT AND GINGER SOUP

This creamy carrot and ginger soup is a filling and satisfying light supper choice. It's created with carrots, ginger, and coconut milk and is thick, creamy, and flavorful.

Ingredients:

1 pound of peeled and sliced carrots

1 chopped onion

2 minced garlic cloves

1 inch of peeled and grated ginger

4 cups veggie broth

1 coconut milk can (14 oz)

Season with salt and pepper to taste.

Instructions:

Warm a drizzle of olive oil in a big saucepan over medium heat

Cook until the onions are transparent and aromatic, then add the garlic and ginger

Bring the diced carrots and vegetable broth to a boil

 Put the heat on low and cook for about 20 minutes, or until the carrots are fluffy or soft

Set aside from the heat and allow to cool

Crush the soup into a thick liquid with an immersion blender

Season with salt and pepper, and stir in the coconut milk

Serve immediately and enjoy!

LENTIL AND VEGETABLE SOUP

Lentil and vegetable soup is a nutritious and nourishing light supper alternative. It's made with lentils, veggies, and spices and is high in protein and fiber.

Ingredients:

1 cup lentils dry

1 chopped onion

2 minced garlic cloves

2 peeled and sliced carrots

2 chopped celery stalks

1 can chopped tomatoes (14 oz)

4 cups veggie broth

1 teaspoon cumin powder

1 teaspoon of coriander powder

Season with salt and pepper to taste.

Instructions:

Warm a drizzle of olive oil in a big saucepan over medium heat

Cook until the onions are transparent and aromatic, then add the garlic and onions

Bring to a boil the chopped carrots, celery, lentils, diced tomatoes, vegetable broth, ground cumin, and ground coriander

Put the heat on low and simmer for about 30 minutes, or until the lentils are well cooked

Season with salt and pepper to taste

Serve immediately and enjoy!

SPINACH AND STRAWBERRY SALAD WITH BALSAMIC VINAIGRETTE

Salad of Spinach and Strawberries with Balsamic Vinaigrette is a light and refreshing supper choice. It's created with fresh spinach, luscious strawberries, and a tart balsamic vinaigrette and is ideal for a hot summer day. Ingredients: 4 cups spinach leaves, fresh 1 cup strawberries, sliced 1 tablespoon balsamic vinaigrette Season with salt and pepper to taste. Instructions: Toss the fresh spinach leaves and cut strawberries in a large mixing dish. Toss with the balsamic vinaigrette to coat. Season with salt and pepper to taste. Serve right away and enjoy!

GRILLED CHICKEN CAESAR SALAD

Grilled chicken Caesar salad is a filling and substantial supper choice. It's a refreshing summer salad prepared with grilled chicken, crisp romaine lettuce, and creamy Caesar dressing.

Ingredients:

1 pound of skinless, boneless chicken breasts

4 cups chopped romaine lettuce

1/4 cup Caesar salad dressing

Season with salt and pepper to taste.

Instructions:

 Preheat the grill to medium-high heat

Add seasoning to both sides of the chicken breasts with pepper and salt

Grill the chicken breasts for 6–8 minutes on each side, or until done

Pull it off the heat and set it aside for about 5 minutes

Chicken breasts should be cut into thin strips

Toss the chopped romaine leaves and cut chicken breasts in a large mixing basin

To coat, drizzle with Caesar dressing

Serve right away and enjoy!

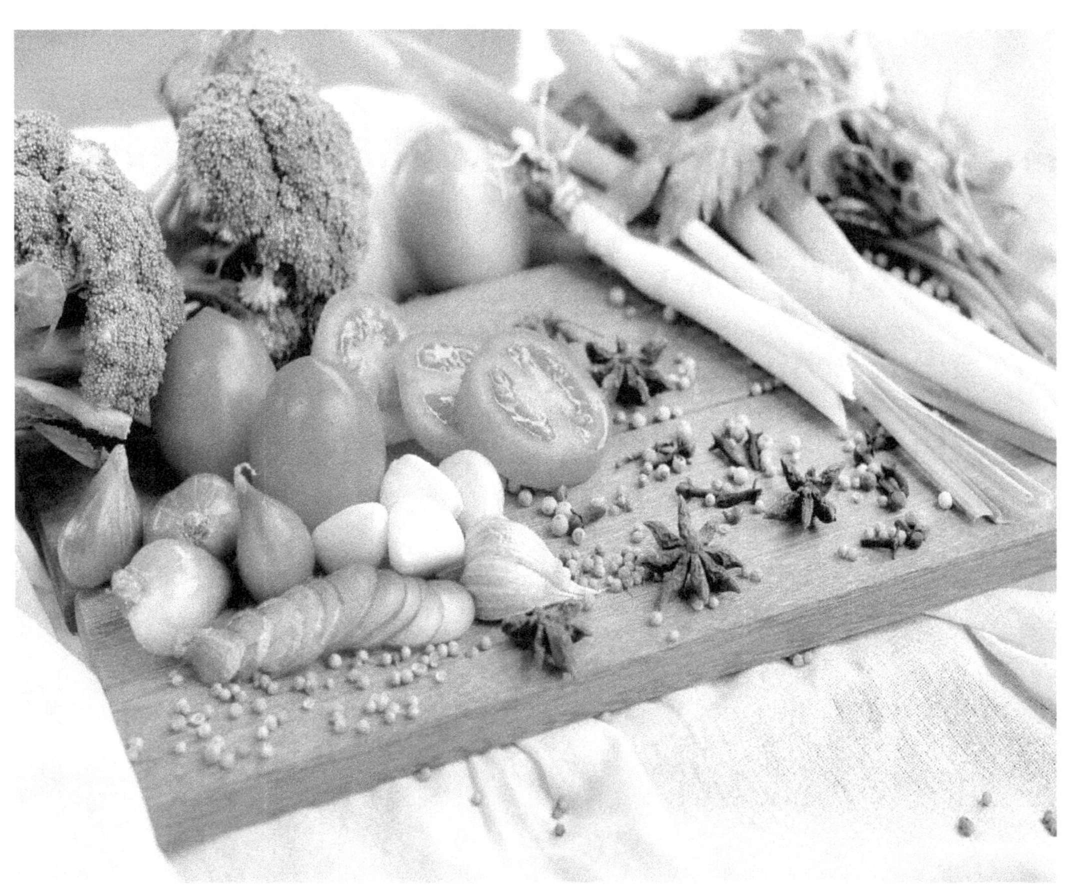

MIXED GREENS SALAD WITH LEMON-TAHINI DRESSING

Lemon-tahini-dressed mixed greens salad is a light and refreshing supper alternative. It's created with mixed greens, cherry tomatoes, and a zesty lemon-tahini dressing that's ideal for a hot summer day.

Ingredients:

4 cups greens mixed

1 cup halved cherry tomatoes

1 tablespoon lemon-tahini dressing

Season with salt and pepper to taste.

Instructions:

Toss the mixed greens and cherry tomatoes in a large mixing basin

Toss with the lemon-tahini dressing to coat

Season with salt and pepper to taste

Serve right away and enjoy!

To summarize, soups and salads are frequently regarded as light and refreshing dinner alternatives, yet they may also be heavy and filling. We've looked at a selection of soup and salad dishes that are not only delicious and savory but also adapted to the specific nutritional needs of people with stage 4 renal disease. These dishes, ranging from creamy carrot and ginger soup to mixed green salad with lemon-tahini dressing, are ideal for a light lunch or a refreshing dinner. So don't put it off any longer.

FIVE

MAIN COURSE RECIPES

When it comes to dinners, the main dish is generally the star of the show, and for good reason. It's the main course—the dish that fills you up and quenches your appetite. However, when you have stage 4 kidney illness, it can be difficult to locate main course selections that are both delicious and kidney-friendly. In this chapter, we'll look at a range of main-course meals that are not only tasty and savory but also customized to the specific dietary requirements of people with stage 4 renal disease. From baked lemon-pepper salmon to stuffed bell peppers with quinoa and black beans, these dishes are sure to delight your taste buds while also leaving you feeling full and content.

BAKED LEMON-PEPPER SALMON

Baked lemon-pepper salmon is a light and tasty main course alternative. It's roasted to perfection in the oven with a simple marinade of lemon juice, olive oil, and black pepper.

Ingredients:

1 pound of salmon fillets

2 tablespoons of olive oil

2 tablespoons of lemon juice

1 teaspoon ground black pepper

Season with salt to taste.

Instructions:

Preheat the oven to 400 degrees Fahrenheit

In a small mixing bowl, combine the olive oil, lemon juice, black pepper, and salt

Drizzle the marinade over the salmon fillets in a baking tray

Bake for 15-20 minutes, or until the salmon flakes easily with a fork

Serve immediately and enjoy!

GRILLED CHICKEN WITH ROASTED VEGETABLES

Grilled chicken with roasted vegetables is a filling and substantial main entrée. It's grilled to perfection and served with roasted veggies, and it's cooked with a simple marinade of olive oil, garlic, and herbs.

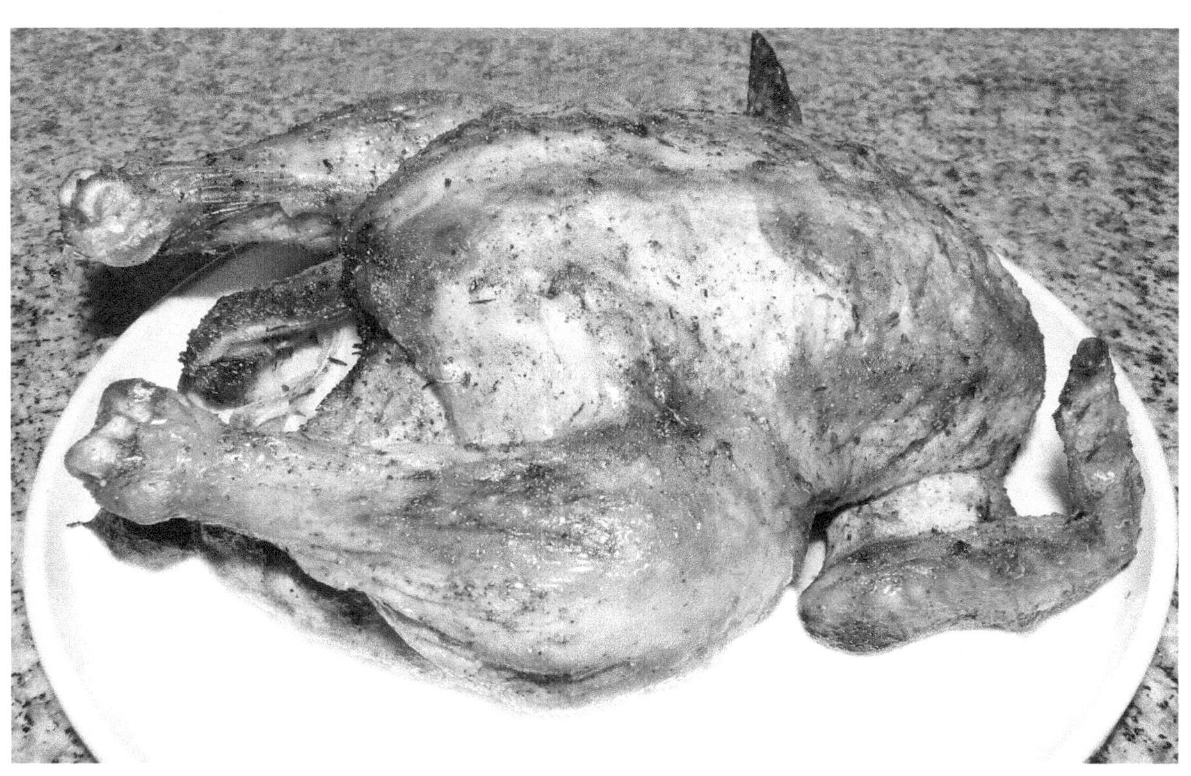

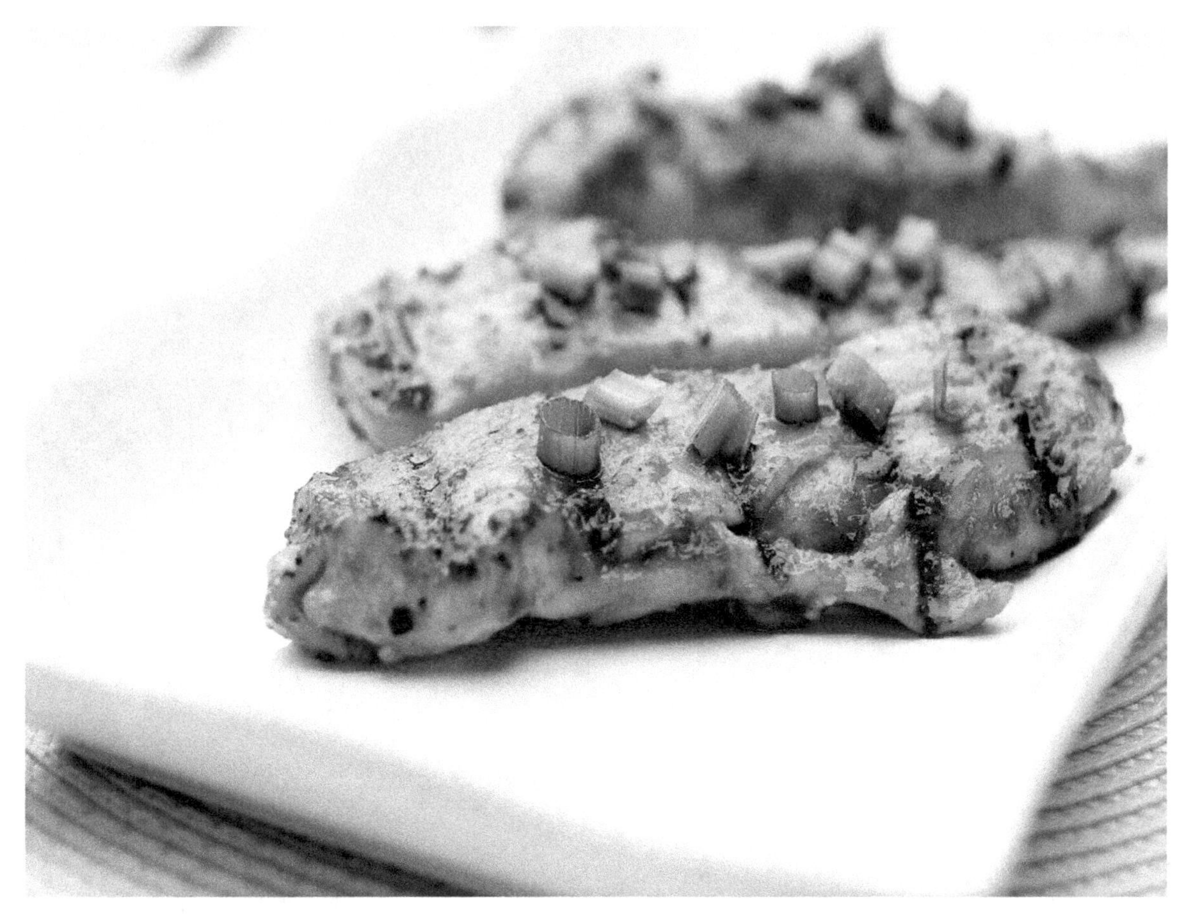

Ingredients:

1 pound of skinless

boneless chicken breasts

2 tablespoons of olive oil

2 minced garlic cloves

1 teaspoon dry herbs (romarino, thyme, or oregano)

Season with salt and pepper to taste

4 cups mixed veggies (bell peppers, zucchini, carrots, etc.)

Instructions:

Whisk together the olive oil, garlic, dried herbs, salt, and pepper in a small bowl

Place the chicken breasts in a resealable plastic bag and drizzle with the marinade

Shake the bag to coat the chicken breasts with the marinade

Allow to marinate for at least 30 minutes, but no more than 24 hours

Preheat the grill to medium-high temperature

Grill the chicken breasts for 6–8 minutes on each side, or until done

Remove from the heat and let it sit for 5 minutes

Preheat the oven to 400°F in the meantime

Drizzle olive oil over the mixed veggies on a baking sheet

Toss to coat, and season with salt and pepper

Roast for 20–25 minutes, or until the vegetables are soft and golden brown

Enjoy the grilled chicken with the roasted veggies!

STIR-FRIED TOFU WITH BROCCOLI AND BELL PEPPERS

Stir-fry tofu with broccoli and bell peppers is a light and tasty main course alternative. It's filled with protein and nutrients and is created with a simple stir-fry sauce of soy sauce, ginger, and garlic.

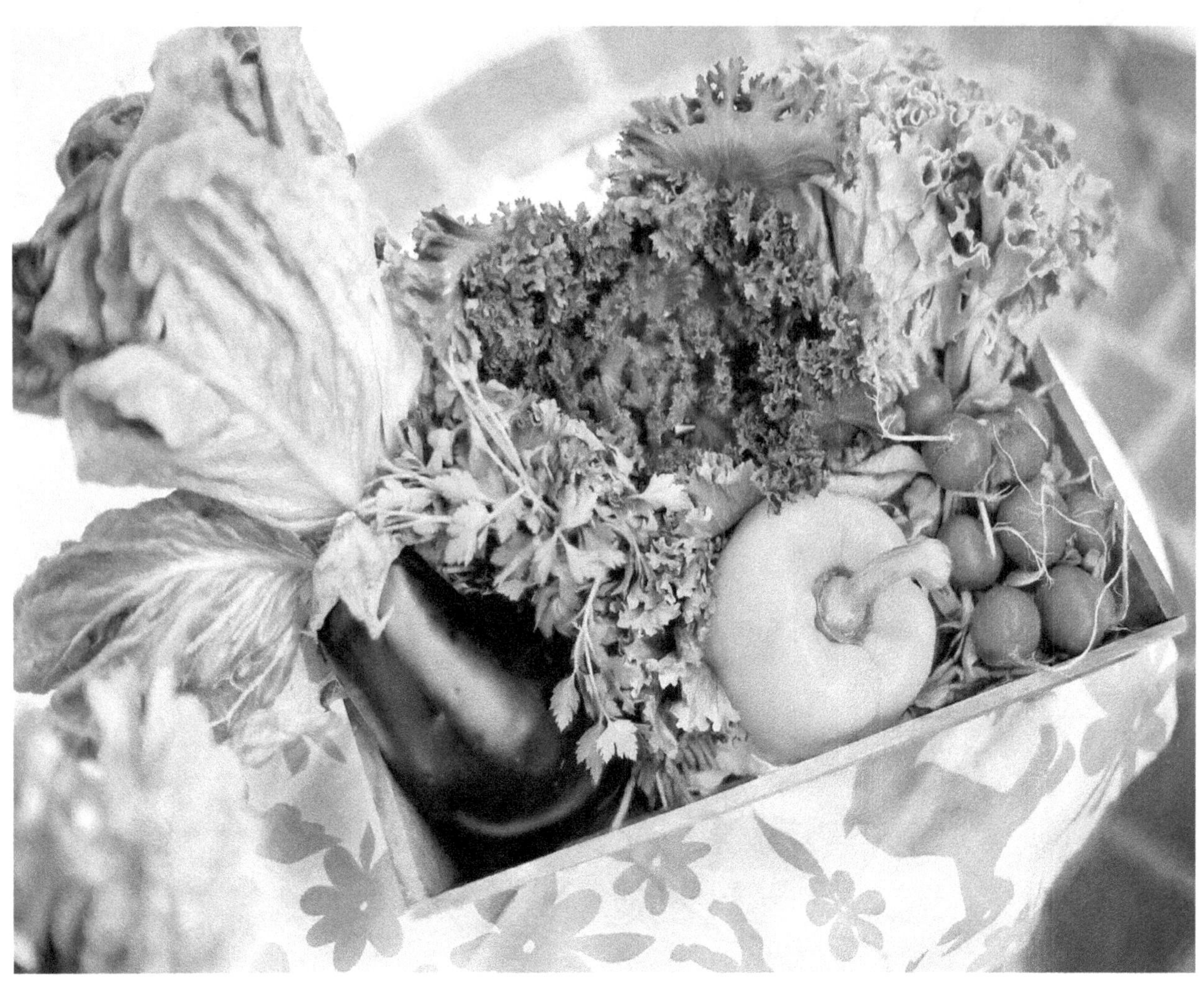

Ingredients:

1 pound of drained and pressed tofu

2 tbsp. of soy sauce

1 teaspoon ginger, grated

2 minced garlic cloves

1 tablespoon extra virgin olive oil

2 cups florets broccoli

1 sliced bell pepper

Season with salt and pepper to taste.

Instructions:

To begin, cut the tofu into cubes and set aside

In a small mixing bowl, combine the soy sauce, grated ginger, and minced garlic

Place the olive oil in a wok or in a large pan over medium-high heat

Cook until the tofu cubes are golden brown and crispy, about 5 minutes

Set the tofu aside after removing it from the pan

Cook until the broccoli florets and bell pepper slices are soft, about 5 minutes

Return the tofu to the pan and drizzle with the stir-fry sauce

Toss to coat and cook for 2 minutes, or until cooked through

Season to taste with salt and pepper

Serve immediately and enjoy!

SLOW-COOKED BEEF STEW

This slow-cooked beef stew is a substantial and comforting main course alternative. It's cooked with soft beef pieces, a variety of veggies, and a savory broth.

Ingredients:

1 pound of cubed beef stew meat

2 tablespoons of olive oil

1 chopped onion

2 minced garlic cloves

4 cups of beef stock

2 peeled and sliced carrots; 2 peeled and sliced potatoes

1 can chopped tomatoes (14 oz)

1 teaspoon dry herbs (romarino, thyme, or oregano)

Season with salt and pepper to taste.

Instructions:

Warm the olive oil in a large saucepan over medium-high heat

Cook until the beef stew meat is browned on both sides

Take the beef out of the saucepan and put it aside

Cook until the onions and garlic are fragrant in the saucepan

Return the meat to the saucepan, along with the beef broth, carrots, potatoes, diced tomatoes, and dry herbs

Bring to a boil, then lower to a low heat and simmer for 2 hours, or until the meat and veggies are cooked

Season to taste with salt and pepper

Serve immediately and enjoy!

QUINOA AND BLACK BEAN STUFFED BELL PEPPERS

Quinoa and Black Bean Stuffed Bell Peppers recipe is a light and tasty main meal. It's created with cooked quinoa, black beans, and veggies, then packed with bell peppers and baked till tender.

Ingredients:

4 big halved and seeded bell peppers

1 cup quinoa, cooked

1 can (14 oz) rinsed and drained black beans

1 cup diced veggies (for example, bell peppers, onions, or tomatoes)

1 teaspoon cumin powder

1 teaspoon of coriander powder

Season with salt and pepper to taste.

Instructions:

Preheat the oven to 400 degrees Fahrenheit

Combine the cooked quinoa, black beans, diced veggies, ground cumin, and ground coriander in a large mixing basin

Toss with salt and pepper until well combined

Fill the halved bell peppers with the mixture and place them on a baking dish

Bake for 30 minutes, covered with foil

Remove the foil and bake for another 10-15 minutes, or until the peppers are soft and the filling is well cooked

Serve immediately and enjoy!

In conclusion, when it comes to meals, the main dish is frequently the star of the show, and choosing delicious and kidney-friendly selections might be difficult. We've looked at a number of major topics in this chapter.

SIX

SIDE DISH RECIPES

Side dishes are frequently the hidden stars of dinners, complementing the main course and adding a layer of taste and texture. However, when you have stage 4 kidney disease, it can be difficult to locate side dishes that are both delicious and kidney-friendly. In this chapter, we'll look at a range of side dishes that are not only tasty and savory but also customized to the specific dietary requirements of people with stage 4 renal disease. From garlic green beans to cilantro-lime rice, these dishes will add a special touch to any meal.

GARLIC GREEN BEANS

These garlic green beans are a quick and easy side dish that is tasty and delicious. They're cooked with a simple blend of green beans, garlic, and olive oil and go great with any main meal.

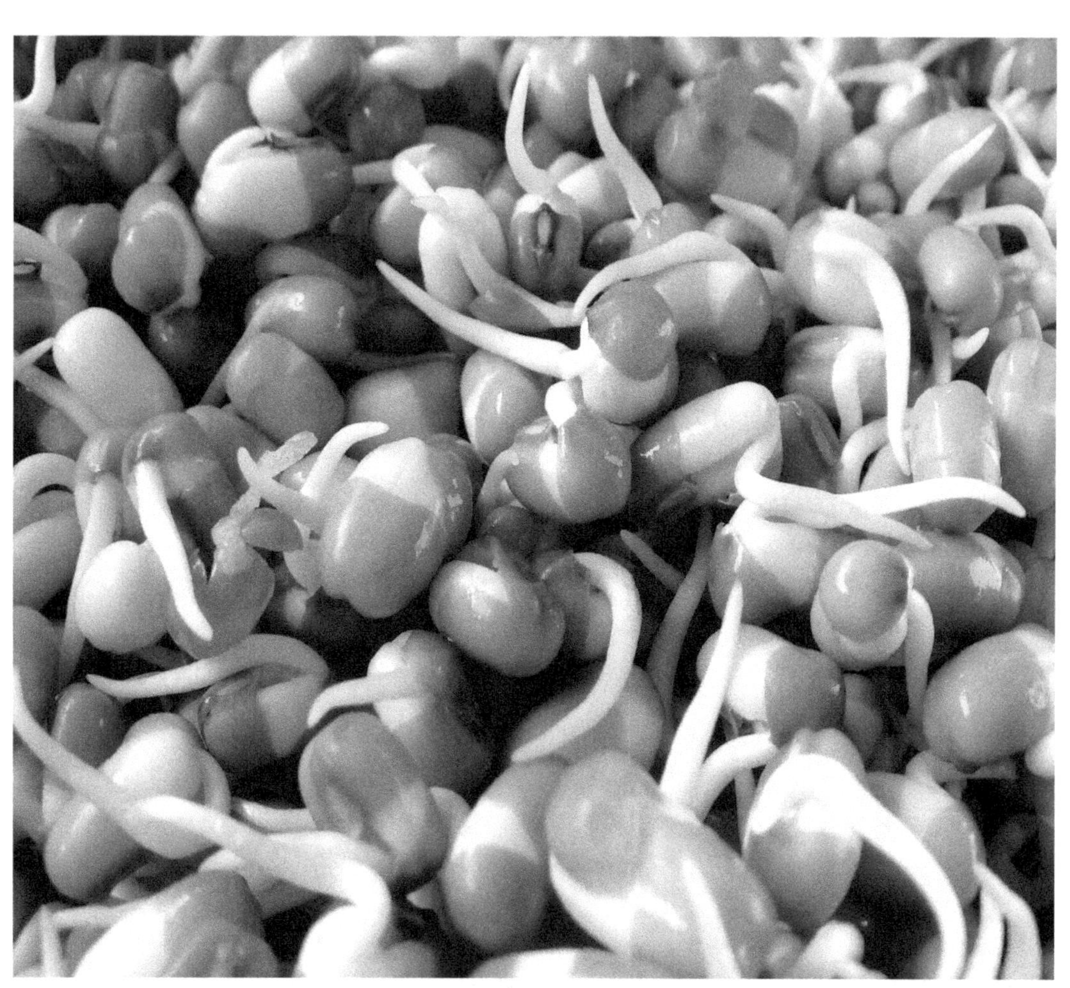

Ingredients:

1 pound of trimmed green beans

2 minced garlic cloves

1 tablespoon extra virgin olive oil

Season with salt and pepper to taste.

Instructions:

Place the olive oil in a large pan over medium heat

Cook until the green beans are tender-crisp, about 5-7 minutes

Cook until the garlic becomes fragrant, for about 1-2 minutes

Season to taste with salt and pepper

Serve immediately and enjoy!

CILANTRO-LIME RICE

Cilantro-lime rice is a refreshing and tasty side dish that is ideal for a summer supper. It's created with a basic blend of rice, cilantro, and lime juice and goes well with any main meal.

Ingredients:

1 cup rice, cooked

2 tbsp. cilantro, chopped

1 teaspoon lime juice

Season with salt and pepper to taste.

Instructions:

Combine the cooked rice, cilantro, and lime juice
in a large mixing basin

Flip or turn to incorporate, and season with
pepper and salt to taste

Serve immediately and enjoy!

ROASTED BRUSSELS SPROUTS

Roasted Brussels sprouts are a substantial and filling side dish that is ideal for a fall supper. They're created with a simple combination of Brussels sprouts, olive oil, and garlic, then roasted in the oven to perfection.

Ingredients:

1 pound of trimmed and halved Brussels sprouts

2 tablespoons of olive oil

2 minced garlic cloves

Season with salt and pepper to taste.

Instructions:

Preheat the oven to 400 degrees Fahrenheit

Toss the Brussels sprouts with the olive oil and minced garlic in a large mixing basin

Season with salt and pepper, and arrange on a baking sheet in a single layer

Between 20 and 25 minutes, or until crispy and golden brown, Serve immediately and enjoy!

MASHED CAULIFLOWER

This mashed cauliflower is a light and creamy side dish ideal for a winter supper. It's created with cauliflower, olive oil, and garlic, and it's mixed to a smooth and creamy texture.

Ingredients:

1 cauliflower head, sliced into florets

2 tablespoons of olive oil

2 minced garlic cloves

Season with salt and pepper to taste.

Instructions:

Bring water to a boil in a big saucepan

Cook until the cauliflower florets are soft, about 15-20 minutes.

Return the cauliflower to the saucepan after draining.

Using an immersion blender, mix in the olive oil and minced garlic until smooth and creamy.

Season to taste with salt and pepper

Serve immediately and enjoy!

GRILLED ASPARAGUS

Grilled asparagus is a quick and easy side dish that is ideal for a summer lunch. It's grilled to perfection with a simple mix of asparagus, olive oil, and garlic.

Ingredients:

1 pound of trimmed asparagus

2 tablespoons of olive oil

2 minced garlic cloves

Season with salt and pepper to taste.

Instructions:

Preheat the grill to medium-high heat

Toss the asparagus with the olive oil and
minced garlic in a large mixing basin

Grill for 5-7 minutes, or until tender and slightly browned, seasoning with salt and pepper

Serve immediately and enjoy!

Finally, side dishes are frequently the unseen heroes of dinners, complementing the main course and giving it an extra layer of taste and texture. We've looked at a selection of side dishes that are not only delicious and savory but also customized to the specific dietary needs of people with stage 4 renal disease.

From garlic green beans to cilantro-lime rice, these dishes will add a special touch to any meal.

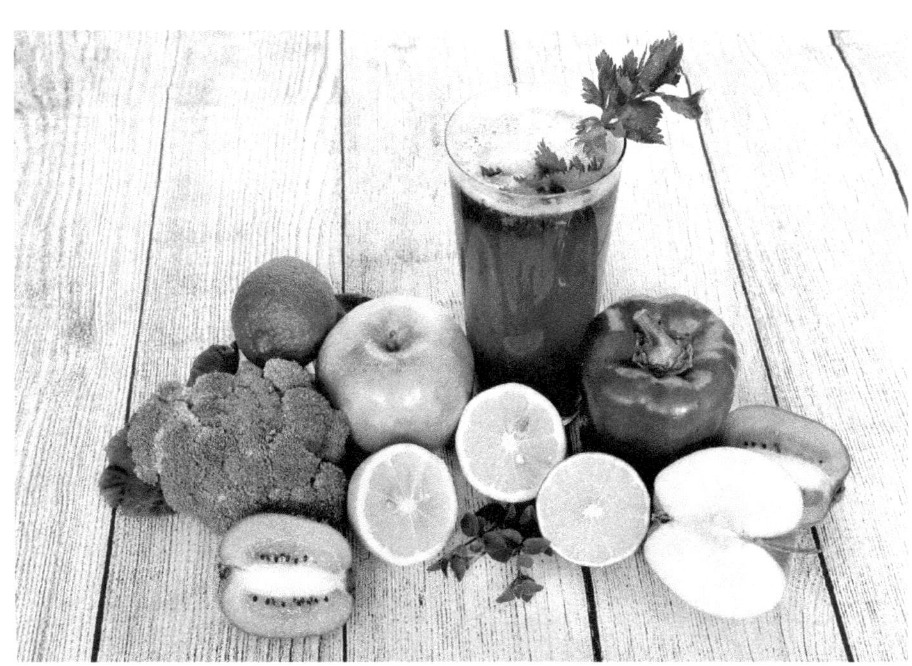

SEVEN

SNACK AND APPETIZER RECIPES

Snacks and appetizers are frequently served as the first course of a dinner, giving a taste of what's to come. They're the ideal method to pique your interest and prepare your taste buds for the main entrée. However, when you have stage 4 kidney disease, it can be difficult to locate snack and appetizer alternatives that are both delicious and kidney-friendly. In this chapter, we'll look at a range of snack and appetizer recipes that are not only tasty and savory but also adapted to the specific dietary needs of people with stage 4 renal disease. These dishes, ranging from roasted chickpeas to stuffed mushrooms, are sure to fulfill your snack needs while leaving you wanting more.

ROASTED CHICKPEAS

Roasted chickpeas are a crispy and tasty snack that is ideal for a mid-day pick-me-up. They're cooked using a simple blend of chickpeas, olive oil, and spices, then baked to perfection.

Ingredients:

1 can (14 oz) of washed and drained chickpeas

2 tablespoons of olive oil

1 teaspoon cumin powder

1 teaspoon of paprika powder

Season with salt and pepper to taste.

Instructions:

Preheat the oven to 400 degrees Fahrenheit

Toss the chickpeas with the olive oil, cumin, paprika, salt, and pepper in a large mixing basin

Roast for 20-25 minutes, or until crispy and golden brown, in a single layer on a baking sheet

Serve immediately and enjoy!

STUFFED MUSHROOMS

Stuffed mushrooms are a flavorful and filling appetizer choice that is ideal for a dinner party or special occasion. They're created with only mushrooms, cream cheese, and herbs, and they're cooked to perfection in the oven.

Ingredients:

12 big mushrooms, removed stems

1 cup softened cream cheese

2 tbsp chopped herbs (parsley, chives, or dill preferred)

Season with salt and pepper to taste.

Instructions:

Preheat the oven to 375 degrees Fahrenheit

In a small mixing dish, combine the cream cheese, chopped herbs, salt, and pepper

Place the mushroom caps on a baking sheet and stuff with the mixture

Bake the mushrooms for 15-20 minutes, or until soft and the filling is golden brown

Serve immediately and enjoy!

GUACAMOLE WITH VEGGIE STICKS

This guacamole with veggie sticks is a light and delicious snack ideal for a hot summer day. It's created with avocados, lime juice, and herbs, and it's served with a variety of vegetable sticks for dipping.

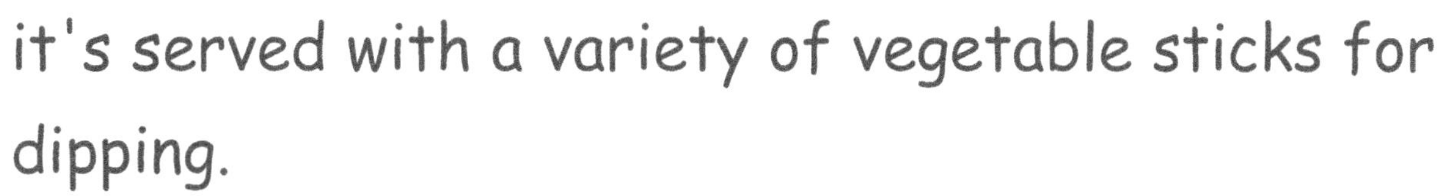

Ingredients:

2 avocados, ripe

1 teaspoon lime juice

2 tbsp chopped herbs (such as cilantro, chives, or dill)

Season with salt and pepper to taste.

Veggie sticks (carrot sticks, cucumber slices, or bell pepper strips, for example)

Instructions:

Mash the avocados with a fork in a small bowl until smooth and creamy

Add the lime juice, herbs, salt, and pepper to taste

Serve with dipping vegetables.

SPICY POPCORN

Spicy popcorn is a tasty and filling snack that's ideal for a movie night or game day. It's created with just popcorn, olive oil, and spices, and it's popped on the stove to perfection.

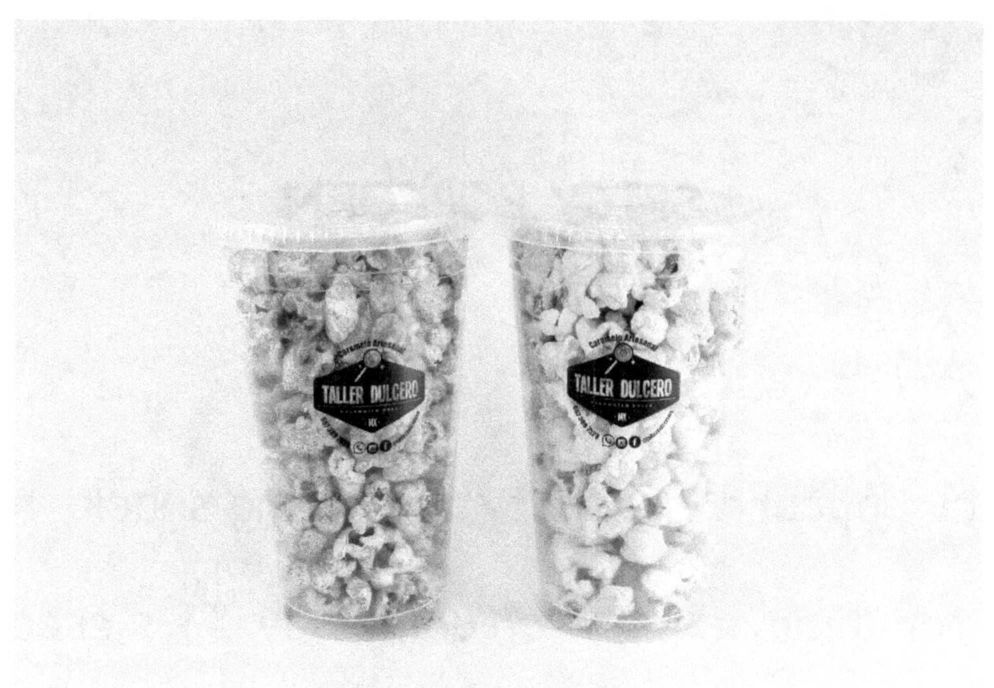

Ingredients:

1 pound of popcorn kernels

2 tablespoons of olive oil

1 teaspoon cumin powder

1 teaspoon of paprika powder

1 tablespoon cayenne pepper

Season with salt and pepper to taste.

Instructions: Warm the olive oil in a large saucepan over medium-high heat

Put a cover over the lid after adding the popcorn kernels

Shake the pot every now and then to keep the popcorn from burning

Remove from heat once the popping has stopped and set aside for 1-2 minutes

Combine the ground cumin, ground paprika, cayenne pepper, salt, and pepper in a small bowl

Toss the popcorn in the spice mixture to coat it

Serve immediately and enjoy!

Finally, nibbles and appetizers are frequently served as the opening course of a dinner, giving a taste of what's to come. We've looked at a selection of snack and appetizer dishes that are not only delicious and savory but also adapted to the specific dietary needs of people with stage 4 renal disease. These dishes, ranging from roasted chickpeas to stuffed mushrooms, are sure to fulfill your snack needs while leaving you wanting more.

EIGHT

DESSERT RECIPES

Dessert is frequently served as the dinner's grand finale, delivering a sweet and gratifying ending to a magnificent meal. Finding dessert alternatives that are both delicious and kidney-friendly might be difficult when you have stage 4 renal disease. In this chapter, we'll look at a range of dessert dishes that are not only tasty and savory but also customized to the specific dietary demands of people with stage 4 renal disease. These dishes, ranging from Berry Parfait to Flourless Chocolate Cake, are sure to fulfill your sweet taste while also leaving you feeling luxurious and pleased.

BERRY PARFAIT

This berry parfait is a light and refreshing dessert that's ideal for a hot summer day. It's prepared with berries, yogurt, and granola, and it's the perfect way to conclude a meal on a sweet note.

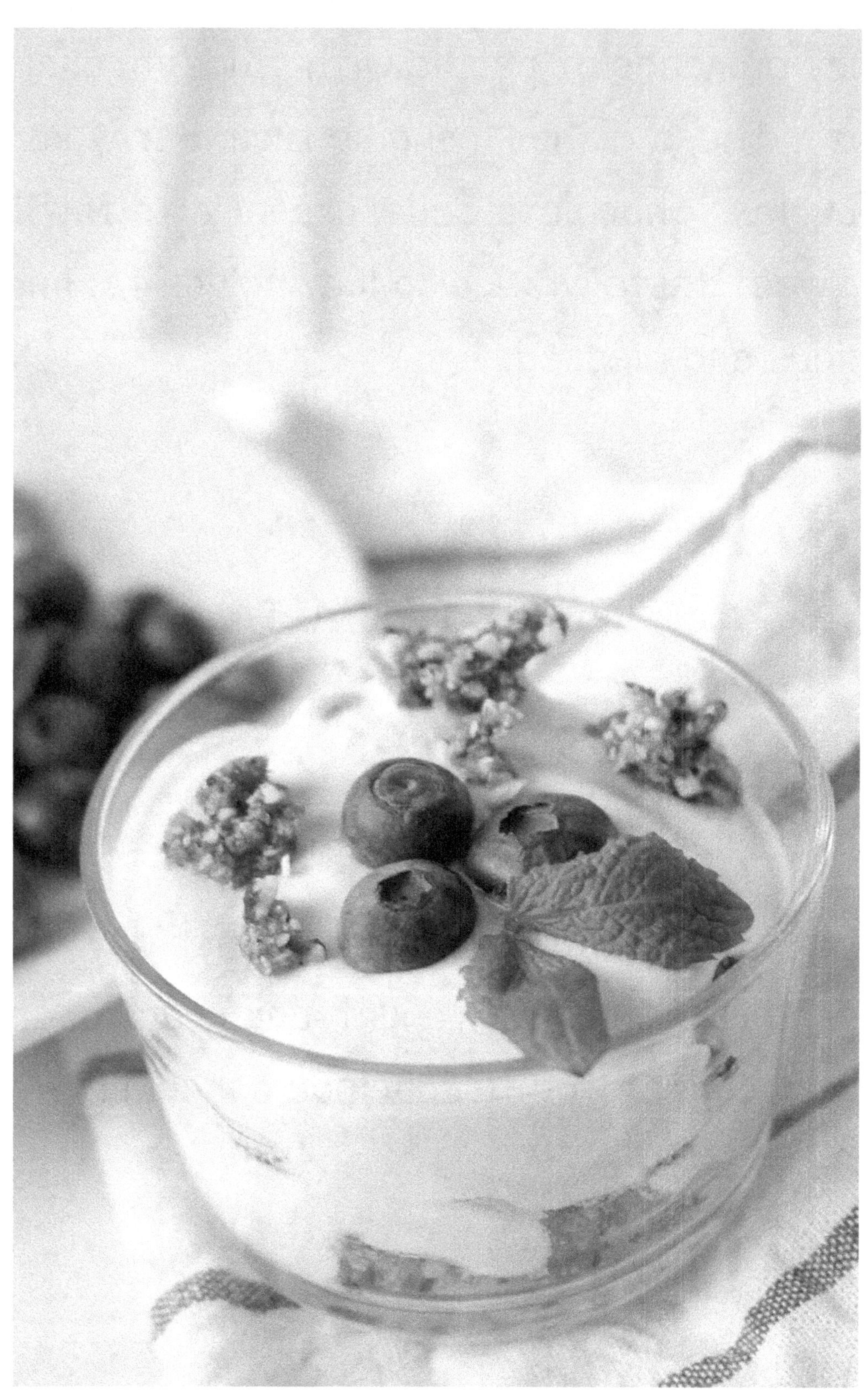

Ingredients:

1 cup mixed berries (strawberries, blueberries, raspberries, etc.)

1 cup plain, low-fat yogurt

2 granola tablespoons Instructions: Layer

1/3 cup yogurt

1/3 cup berries

1 tablespoon granola in a glass or container

Continue layering until all of the ingredients are used

Serve right away and enjoy!

FLOURLESS CHOCOLATE CAKE

Flourless chocolate cake is a rich and decadent dessert ideal for a special occasion. It's created with just three ingredients: chocolate, eggs, and sugar, and it's cooked to perfection in the oven.

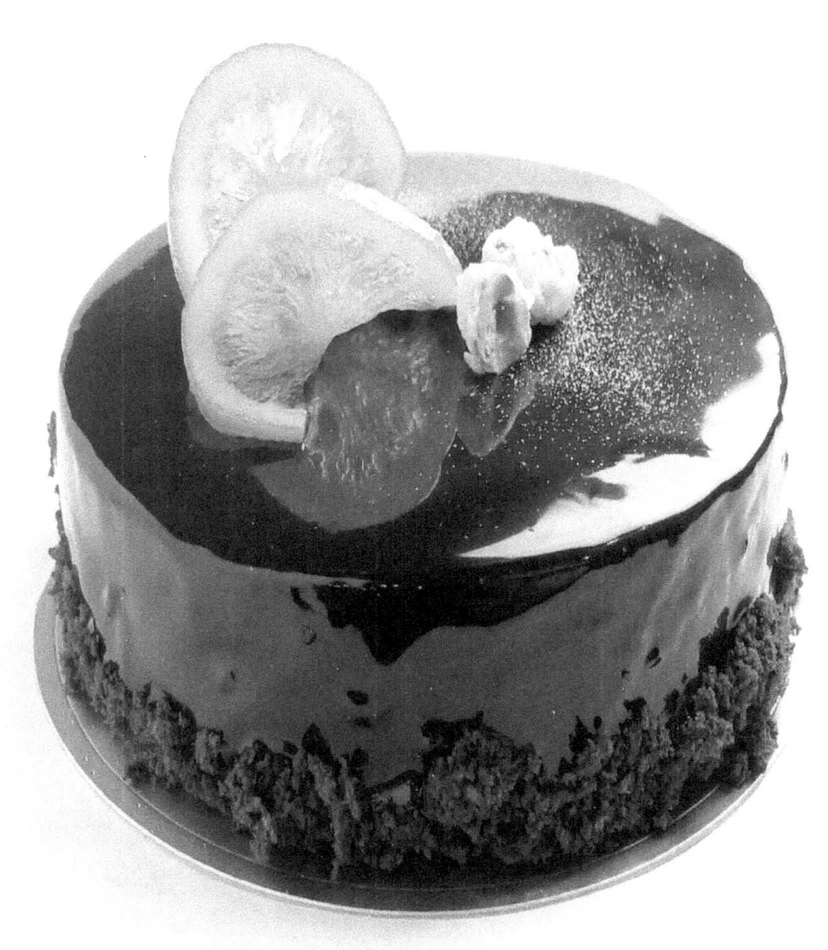

Ingredients:

6 ounces of chopped dark chocolate

1 pound unsalted butter

granulated sugar, 3/4 cup

a quarter teaspoon of salt, and a teaspoon of vanilla extract three huge eggs

a half-cup cocoa powder

Instructions:

Preheat the oven to 375°F and oil an 8-inch round cake pan with cooking spray

Melt the chocolate and butter in a heatproof dish over a saucepan of boiling water

Take the pan off the heat and mix in the sugar, salt, and vanilla extract

Add the eggs one after the other, mixing thoroughly after each addition

Fold in the chocolate powder until barely blended

Smooth the top of the batter into the prepared pan

Bake for 20-25 minutes, or until a toothpick inserted into the middle yields a few moist crumbs

Allow to cool for 10 minutes in the pan before transferring to a wire rack to cool fully

Serve and have fun!

PEACH AND ALMOND TART

Peach and almond tart is a light and flavorful dessert ideal for a hot summer day. It's created with just peaches, almonds, and honey, and it's cooked to perfection in the oven.

Ingredients:

1 cup almond flour

1 tablespoon granulated sugar

a quarter teaspoon of salt

4 tablespoons melted unsalted butter

2 pitted and sliced ripe peaches

2 teaspoons of honey

Instructions:

Preheat the oven to 350°F and coat a 9-inch tart
pan with cooking spray

In a large mixing basin, combine the almond meal,
sugar, and salt

Mix in the melted butter until completely mixed

 Press the mixture into the prepared pan's
bottom and up the edges

Drizzle with honey, and arrange the peach slices on top of the crust

Cook for 20-25 minutes, or until the crust is golden brown and the peaches are soft

Allow to cool for 10 minutes in the pan before transferring to a wire rack to cool fully

Serve and have fun!

LEMON SORBET

Lemon sorbet is a light and tart dessert that is ideal for a hot summer day. It's created with just lemon juice, sugar, and water, then churned to perfection in an ice cream machine.

Ingredients:

1 granulated sugar cup

1 cup of water

1 cup freshly squeezed lemon juice

1 teaspoon of lemon zest

Instructions:

Combine the sugar and water in a small saucepan and cook over medium heat until the sugar is dissolved

Take it off the heat and allow it to cool. Mix in the lemon juice and zest

Fill an ice cream maker halfway with the mixture and churn according to the manufacturer's directions

Transfer to a freezer-safe container and freeze for 2 hours, or until hard

Serve and have fun!

Finally, dessert is frequently the big climax of a dinner, offering a sweet and gratifying ending to a good meal. We've looked at a selection of dessert recipes that are not only tasty and savory but also customized to the specific dietary demands of people with stage 4 renal disease. These dishes, ranging from Berry Parfait to

Flourless Chocolate Cake, are sure to fulfill your sweet taste while also leaving you feeling luxurious and pleased.

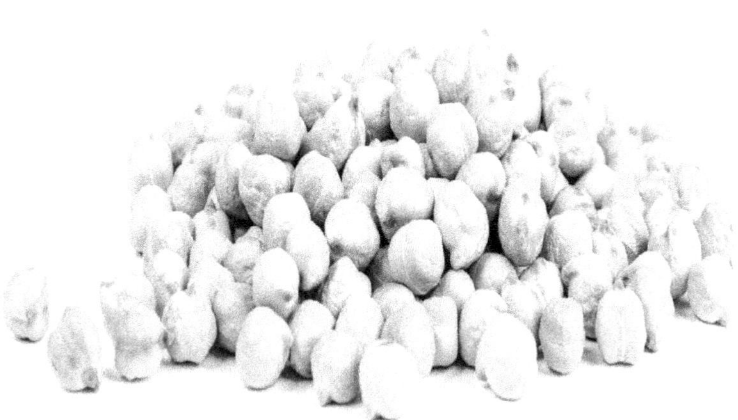

NINE

TIPS FOR HEALTHY EATING WITH STAGE 4 KIDNEY DISEASE

Living with stage 4 kidney disease may be difficult, especially when it comes to eating correctly. A kidney-friendly diet is critical for disease management and delaying progression. In this chapter, we'll look at some suggestions and methods for eating healthy with stage 4 kidney disease, such as how to pick the correct foods, make meals more kidney-friendly, and maintain a balanced and nutritious diet.

UNDERSTANDING KIDNEY-FRIENDLY FOODS

Understanding which foods are kidney-friendly and which to avoid is the first step toward healthy eating with stage 4 renal disease. A kidney-friendly diet is high in protein and fiber and low in salt, phosphorus, and potassium. Fruits and vegetables, whole grains, lean meats, and healthy fats are all examples of kidney-friendly diets. Meals rich in salt, phosphorus, and potassium, such as processed meals, fast foods, and high-potassium fruits and vegetables, on the other hand, should be limited or avoided.

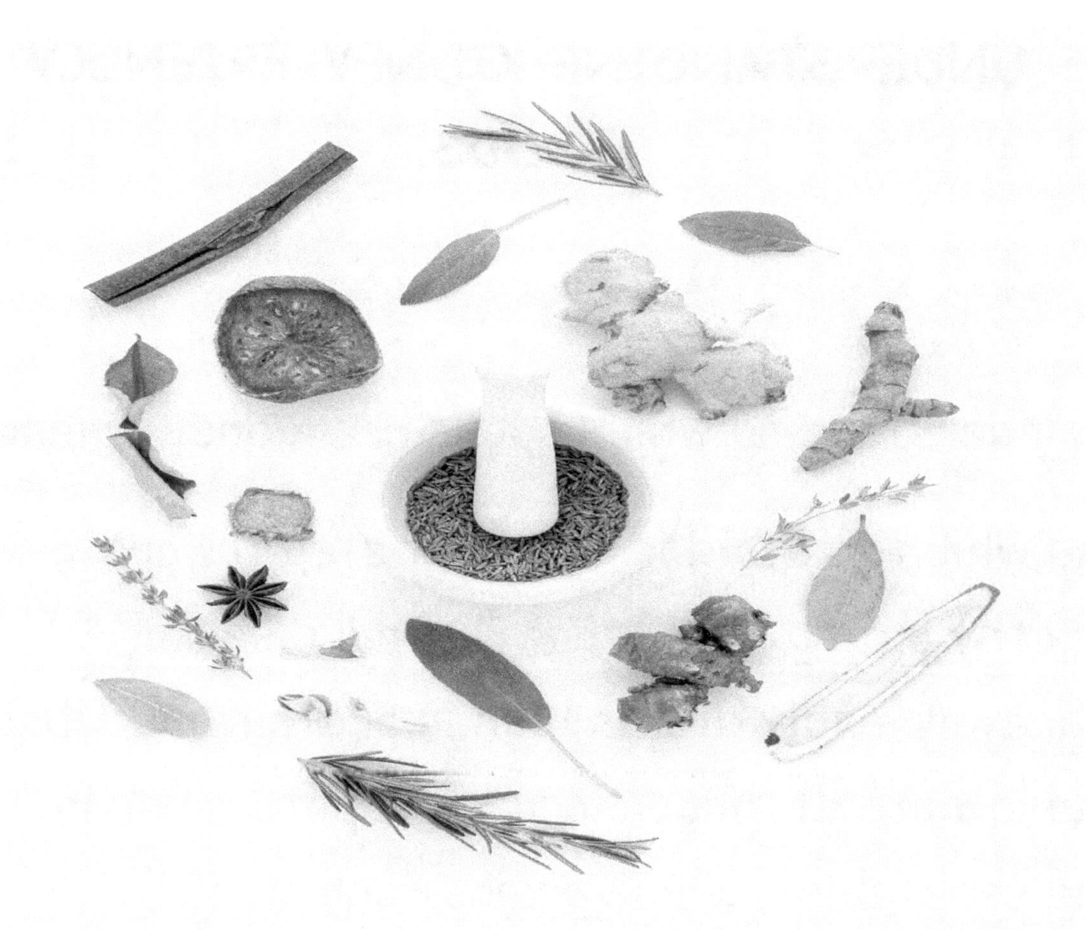

PLANNING AND PREPARING MEALS

Once you've determined which foods are kidney-friendly, the next step is to plan and prepare meals that are both tasty and healthy. This can be difficult, especially if you're accustomed to eating in a specific manner. However, with a little imagination and organization, you can prepare meals that are not only excellent for your kidneys but also enjoyable and filling. Here are some ideas for planning and cooking kidney-friendly meals:

Select lean proteins: Lean proteins, such as chicken, turkey, fish, and tofu, are high in protein while being low in phosphorus and salt. When feasible, add lean proteins to your meals.

Fresh or frozen fruits and vegetables are low in salt and phosphorus and are a terrific way to add taste and nutrients to your meals. Rich-potassium foods should be restricted or avoided. Some fruits and vegetables, such as bananas, oranges, and potatoes, are rich in potassium and should be limited or avoided.

Choose low-potassium fruits and vegetables like apples, berries, and carrots instead. Keep an eye out for hidden salt. Processed foods, quick foods, and restaurant meals are frequently high in sodium, so avoid them as much as possible. Cook at home instead, using fresh or frozen ingredients.

Make a plan: Meal planning can help you make better choices and avoid last-minute temptations. Plan your meals for the week and create a shopping list to ensure you have everything you need.

MAINTAINING A BALANCED AND NUTRITIOUS DIET

Finally, it's critical to eat a well-balanced, healthy diet tailored to your specific needs. Because we are different and unique from one another, what works for some people may not work for others. Create a tailored meal plan with a qualified dietitian or a healthcare expert that suits your individual requirements and objectives. Here are some suggestions for eating a well-balanced and healthy diet:

Keep track of your nutritional consumption. Track your salt, phosphorus, and potassium intake to verify you're keeping within the suggested levels. Drink plenty of water. Water is essential for kidney function and general health. Unless your healthcare physician advises differently, aim for at least 8 glasses of water every day.

Limit added sugars: Sugary beverages, sweets, and baked products with added sugars can lead to weight gain and other health concerns. When feasible, try to restrict your intake of added sugars.

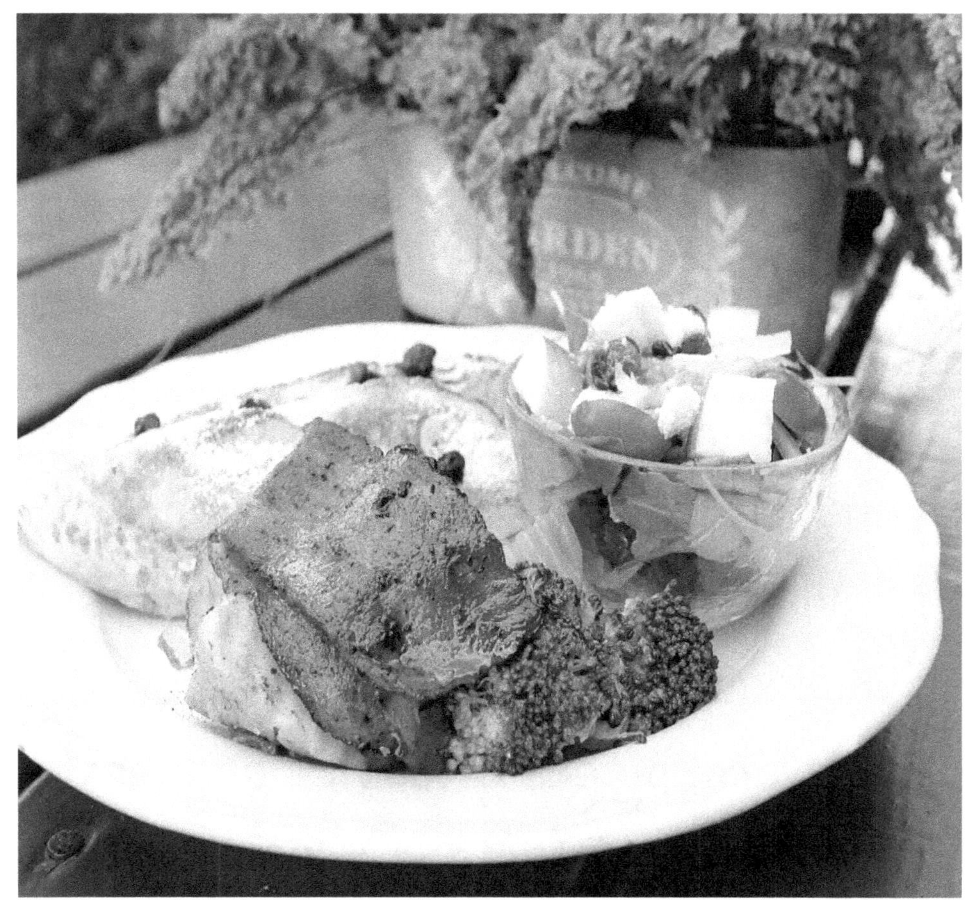

Select whole grains: Whole grains, such as brown rice, quinoa, and whole wheat bread, are high in fiber and minerals that are beneficial to your kidneys and general health. Include healthy fats. Healthy fats, such as those found in avocados, almonds, and olive oil, are essential for heart health and overall well-being. When feasible, add healthy fats to your diet.

To summarize, living with stage 4 kidney disease is difficult, but with the correct tactics and support, you can make good eating choices that benefit your kidneys and overall health. We've looked at several pieces of advice and methods for healthy eating with stage 4 kidney disease, such as how to pick the proper foods, make meals more kidney-friendly, and maintain a balanced and nutritious diet.

TEN

SAMPLE MEAL PLANS FOR STAGE 4 KIDNEY DISEASE

Creating a meal plan that is both delicious and kidney-friendly can be difficult, especially if you have stage 4 kidney disease. However, with a little imagination and organization, you can prepare meals that are not only excellent for your kidneys but also enjoyable and filling. In this chapter, we'll look at some sample meal plans for stage 4 renal disease that are adapted to the specific dietary requirements of those suffering from this condition. These meal plans are designed to give you the nutrition you require while keeping your kidneys healthy from breakfast to supper.

SAMPLE MEAL PLAN 1

Breakfast:

whole grain bread and scrambled eggs with spinach Salad with fresh fruits

Lunch: Salad with grilled chicken, mixed greens, cherry tomatoes, and vinaigrette dressing
Stuffed bell peppers with quinoa and black beans

Dinner: Lemon-pepper salmon baked in the oven with roasted Brussels sprouts and mashed cauliflower

Snack: chickpeas roasted

Dessert: Fruit parfait

SAMPLE MEAL PLAN 2

Breakfast: Greek yogurt topped with granola and fresh fruit Sliced oranges

Lunch: Wrap with turkey and avocado, whole grain tortilla, lettuce, and tomato Hummus on carrot and celery sticks

Dinner: Grilled shrimp over cilantro lime rice, with grilled asparagus

Snack: almond butter with apple slices

Dessert: chocolate cake made without flour

SAMPLE MEAL PLAN 3

Breakfast: sliced almonds, honey, and fresh fruit on oatmeal, halved grapefruit

Lunch: Salad with tuna, mixed greens, cherry tomatoes, and a lemon vinaigrette dressing Cheese on whole grain crackers

Dinner: Tofu stir-fried with broccoli and bell peppers Green beans with garlic

Snack: popcorn with a spicy kick

Dessert: tart with peaches and almonds

To summarize, developing a meal plan that is both pleasant and kidney-friendly might be difficult, but with a little imagination and forethought, you can design meals that are not only excellent for your kidneys but also enjoyable and gratifying. This chapter has looked at several sample meal plans for stage 4 renal disease that are customized to the specific dietary demands of people with this illness.

CONCLUSION

To summarize, living with stage 4 kidney disease can be difficult, but with the correct information, tools, and support, you can regain control of your health and well-being. This cookbook is intended to give you tasty and nutrient-dense dishes that are adapted to the specific dietary demands of people with stage 4 renal disease. These meals, from breakfast to dessert, are not only excellent for your kidneys but also flavorful and enjoyable.

We hope that this cookbook has motivated you to take control of your health and make positive dietary and lifestyle changes. Remember that every modest step you take toward greater health and well-being is a positive step. So don't put it off any longer. Begin experimenting in the kitchen and take the first step toward a healthier and happier future.

Thank you for your interest in "The Stage 4 Kidney Protector Cookbook." On your road to improved health and happiness, we wish you the greatest of health and happiness. Your health is important to us, and we're here to help you every step of the way.

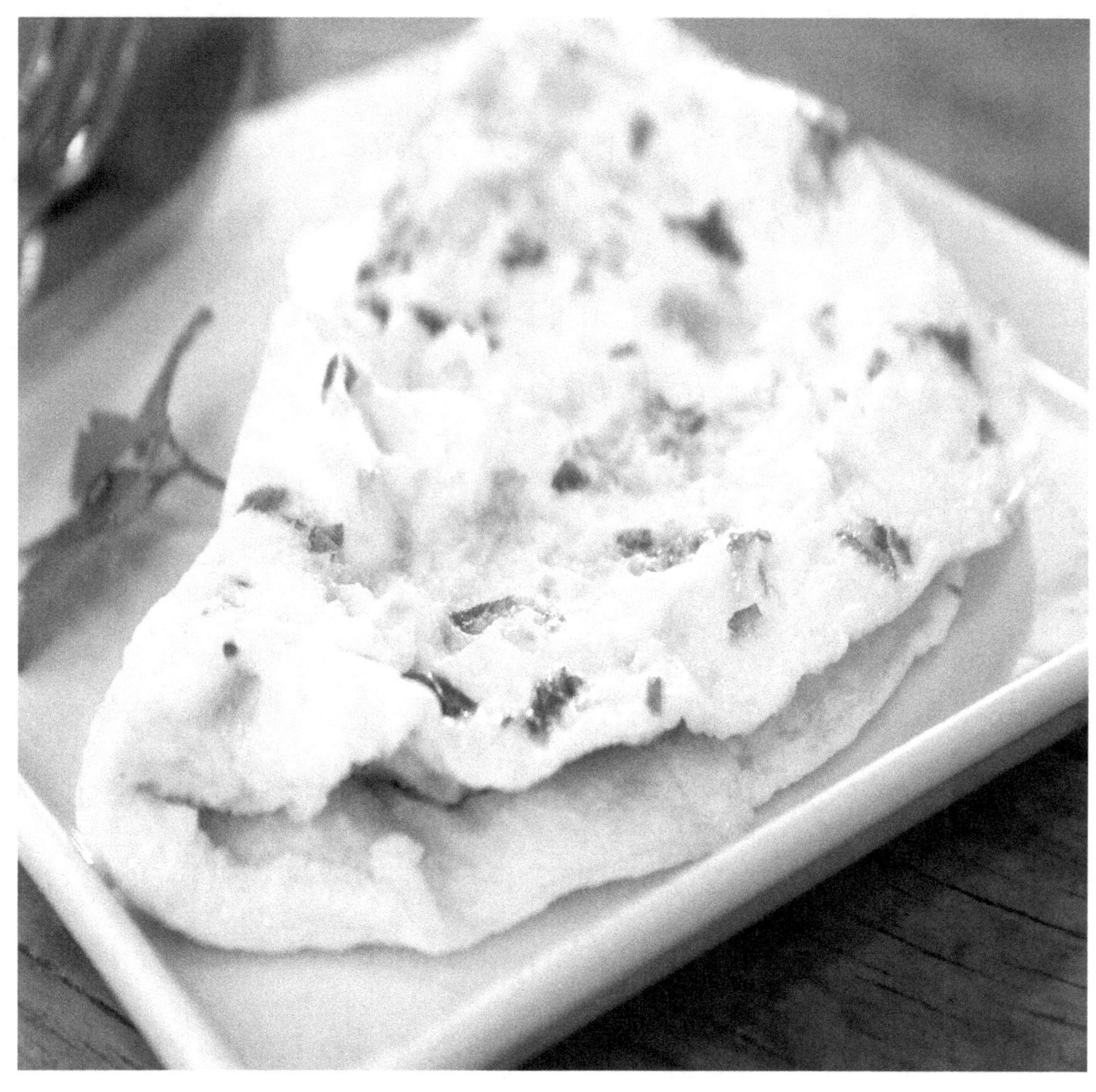

For more information and helpful tips on health, diet and fitness, cookbook, wine and food recipes. Click here

https://www.amazon.com/author/shauverivk